I0406994

Epsom Salt:

20 Amazing Secrets How To Use This Magnesium-Rich Miracle For Your Beauty And Health

All photos used in this book, including the cover photo were made available under a Attribution-NonCommercial-ShareAlike 2.0 Generic and sourced from Flickr

Copyright 2016 by the publisher - All rights reserved.

This document is geared towards providing exact and reliable information in regards to the topic and issue covered. The publication is sold with the idea that the publisher is not required to render accounting, officially permitted, or otherwise, qualified services. If advice is necessary, legal or professional, a practiced individual in the profession should be ordered.

- From a Declaration of Principles which was accepted and approved equally by a Committee of the American Bar Association and a Committee of Publishers and Associations.

In no way is it legal to reproduce, duplicate, or transmit any part of this document in either electronic means or in printed format. Recording of this publication is strictly prohibited and any storage of this document is not allowed unless with written permission from the publisher. All rights reserved.

The information provided herein is stated to be truthful and consistent, in that any liability, in terms of inattention or otherwise, by any usage or abuse of any policies, processes, or directions contained within is the solitary and utter responsibility of the recipient reader. Under no circumstances will any legal responsibility or blame be held against the publisher for any reparation, damages, or monetary loss due to the information herein, either directly or indirectly.

Respective authors own all copyrights not held by the publisher.

The information herein is offered for informational purposes solely, and is universal as so. The presentation of the information is without contract or any type of guarantee assurance.

The trademarks that are used are without any consent, and the publication of the trademark is without permission or backing by the trademark owner. All trademarks and brands within this book are for clarifying purposes only and are the owned by the owners themselves, not affiliated with this document.

Table of content

Introduction

There you are, browsing another health and beauty section in another department store. You pace back and forth, looking at shelf after shelf, reading label after label, looking for that one thing that is going to solve all of your health and beauty issues.

You read this lotion which claims to hold the secret to what you need. You browse that cream that promises exactly the cure you are looking for. You see that pill that tells you everything you want to hear, and exactly how you are going to be perfected through using the product.

But you can't help but sit back and wonder how effective these things really are. How do you know they are going to work? How do you know they are going to do what they say they are going to do? How do you know they are going to fix your issues and give you that healthy life they are promising?

All of these questions come flooding through your mind, and you are left with your head spinning, always wondering if they are really going to work like they say. The fact of the matter is, they probably aren't going to. You are going to spend all your time and money on things that don't really work, always in the quest to find the one thing that does.

So what do you do? Do you give up? Is it time you tossed in the towel and let it all go?

You may be wondering the same thing. But listen... now is not the time.

You have finally found the book that is going to give you the answers you have been seeking, and show you that you don't have to use pills and products to become the best version of yourself. All you need is the right kind of cure... and that is what I am going to give you.

With this book, you are going to get exactly what you are after, all without the products they try to convince you to get at the stores. I am going to show you the miracle cure you need, and show you how to use it

So if you are ready to toss all those lotions and creams and start doing things the all natural... and truly effective way, you have come to the right place.

Let's get started.

Chapter 1 – Epsom Salt: An Overview

Salt. You are well aware of this little mineral I'm sure. Whether you think of it as the perfect seasoning to any dinner, the age old preservative that has stood the test of time, or that little menace that is responsible for high blood pressure, you are aware of what salt is.

But what you may not know, is that Epsom salt is not the same as the table salt you are thinking of. No, it's not just some distant larger cousin. In fact, Epsom salt is actually a mineral known as magnesium sulfate.

Magnesium sulfate is a pure mineral with countless uses. For centuries, it has been used by people around the world for more reasons than you could even begin to guess. In fact, to this day doctors, athletes, naturalists, and dozens of people in between swear by this rich mineral and everything it can do.

I'm sure you have heard of people recommending using salts for bathing long before now. Surely you have even heard the recommendation of Epsom salt, and listened to the countless tales of all the things it can do for you.

But, what few people actually address, and what you may be wondering is *why* it works the way that it does. Let me explain.

As I said, Epsom salt isn't really salt at all, but rather a mineral which is known as Magnesium sulfate.

Magnesium sulfate has long been known to treat a long range of illnesses including:

- Aches and pains

- Stiffness

- Infections

- Muscle tension

- Nerve tension

- Pressure points

- Nausea

- Poor circulation

- Blood clots

- Thickening arteries

- And more

As you can see by this list alone, there are many, many things this mineral treats. But, this isn't a complete list, as there are plenty of people who stand by the fact it also helps the body with insulin management, constipation, upset stomach, or even mental issues such as anxiety or insomnia.

Though it may appear to be only a mineral on the outside, using this mineral often is going to change your life like you couldn't imagine. But you don't just have to take my word for it.

Let's get you started on your own Epsom salt routine. I want to find a way to bring it into your life on a daily basis. If you don't like it, don't stick with it, but trust me, it's not going to take long before you are hooked for good.

It is my goal with this book to show you just how many ways you can use Epsom salt in your day, whether it's through beauty and health routines, cleaning routines, or just in ways you never thought of before.

There's a reason this has been around for centuries, and why so many professionals in many different fields still recommend it to this day. I am going to show you some of the best ways to use Epsom salt, and how you can cure or relieve virtually any issue in your day.

And, if you want to throw in added benefits, go with the essential oils. They are all natural, easy to find, and the benefits blend seamlessly with those from the Epsom salts. There's no end to the combinations you can make, and no end to the ways you can use natural remedies for the relief you need.

Dive into this book with an open mind, and get ready to feel the relief start to roll in. Trust me, I know what it's like to need relief, and to need it now, and I have tried each and every one of the methods I am going to recommend to you in this book. They are here because they work, and I recommend them to you because I want you to have the same relief that I do, no matter what it is you are dealing with.

Get ready to change your life with just a little miracle mineral you haven't thought of using before, and get rid of all that stress and tension that has tried to build up. With this book, you have it all. The good, the great, and the best of the best.

So, let's not waste any more time... you know you are dying to get the secret to your unlimited health and beauty, and that is the very thing I am going to give you. Let's get started.

Chapter 2 – Legendary Secrets of Epsom Salt Part 1: The Health and the Beauty

You want it all. Excellent health, beautiful skin. Energy to do the things you want to do, and no pain to hold you back. Skin that is soft and hair that is thick, texturized, and shiny.

When you are dealing with the real world, you have to pick and choose what you get, or you have to spend an arm and a leg on all the different products to fill in the gaps of what the others leave out.

But, when you decide to use Epsom salt, you are going to get the best of both worlds, and not have to worry about the negative added chemicals and ingredients they like to slip into those products at the store. Get ready to dive into a whole new way of doing things... be careful, you won't want to go back.

Overall Health Soak

This is a very well-known method, and one that you may have tried in the past, but no Epsom salt book is complete without it. Add 1 cup of Epsom salt the next time you are soaking in a warm bath.

This is good for:

- All over body relaxation
- Increases circulation

- Ache and pain reduction

Splinter Remover

You don't have to go all in to enjoy the benefits of Epsom salt, in fact, just soaking a single part of your body in this mineral is going to help you gain incredible benefits.

If you have a splinter, try adding ¼ cup Epsom salt to a bowl of warm water, and soak your affected area in the bath. Within minutes, it's going to pull the splinter to the surface.

Rub a Dub Scrub

Not only can you use Epsom salt to absorb extra minerals into your body, but you can rid your body of dry skin while you do it. Blend 1 cup Epsom salt with 2 tablespoons coconut oil, and the essential oil of your choice (optional, of course) and scrub your hands and feet in it next time you are in the tub.

Not only are you going to soak in the benefits of the mineral (and any essential oil you decide to use), but you are going to scrub off all the dry skin from your hands and feet and be left with super soft skin.

Don't forget the facial

Who says your hands and feet are the only ones who get to enjoy the rich benefits of this scrub? Try adding a teaspoon to your face soap the next time you are lathering up, and you will feel the tingling warmth of its exfoliating power.

Not to mention you will soak up some of the wonderful benefits as you scrub, a complete win all around if you ask me.

Texture Anyone?

You could go to your local department store and spend your hard earned money on the texturizing sea salt spray they sell these days, or you could add 2 teaspoons to your own spray bottle and enjoy the same benefits at home for a fraction of the cost.

Not only are you going to get that insane texture everyone is ranting about, but you are going to also do your hair some good by avoiding the chemicals and added ingredients they sneak into those products at the store.

This is going to give you that boost you want with none of the negative side effects.

And these are just a few of the rich benefits you are going to get from using this salt. In the chapters to come, we are going to dive deeper into lesser known qualities of this salt... you may even be surprised.

Chapter 3 – Dealing with Issues Only Skin Deep

All women love to do things to make themselves pretty. It's something that has been born into everyone from the beginning of mankind. But, few women realize just how much they can do with the natural things around them, and instead choose to spend a lot of money on products at the store what end up doing more harm than good.

In this chapter, I am going to show you all of the ways you can use Epsom salt in your beauty routine, and end up with hair, skin, and nails that are far better than anything you could achieve from using products you get at the store.

Are you ready? You deserve some pampering time, so grab your Epsom salt and a magazine and sit back and relax. The results are going to blow your mind.

Give yourself the all day spa treatment at home

Any one of us would jump at the chance to go spend the day at the spa, soaking up the goodness in the steam room and melting our problems away in the pool. But, most of us live in the real world and it's just not feasible to get to spend days at the spa.

That's why you have to do things to bring the spa home. And with Epsom salt, you can do that very thing. Mix 2 cups Epsom salt with 1 teaspoon lavender essential oil and add to your warm bath. Soak for as long as you like, and let all the toxins rush out of your body while you soak in the richness of the mineral.

Add body and shine to your mane

Not only does Epsom salt add texture to your hair, by adding a teaspoon to your shampoo, you are going to give both shine and volume to your hair as well. Give yourself the royal treatment at least a couple times a week for the best results, and let your mane free!

Create the best (gentle) salt scrub for your dry lips

Winter is one of the hardest times of year for the skin. The air gets dry and it seems all the moisture in your skin goes right along with it. But, not many people know that they can remove this dry, cracked skin from their lips and replace it with smooth, fresh skin beneath.

With a little bit of Epsom salt mixed with just a dab of coconut oil, you have the perfect scrub for your lips. Apply a little on your finger and gently brush it over your lips, massaging it in and around.

Be gently, your lips are sensitive, and you don't want to be too harsh. Rinse off with warm water and finish with a bit of chapstick, and say hello to your soft, new lips!

Bring permanent volume and health to your hair

Texture is one thing, and a boost of body and shine is another, but who can say no to all day volume? With this treatment, your hair is going to stand tall for as long as you want it to, and be healthier, too.

Simply mix equal parts Epsom salt with your favorite conditioner and massage it all through your hair, focusing more on your hair than your scalp. Sit back and relax as it sits in your hair for 20 minutes, then rinse thoroughly.

Enjoy the insane volume and shine all day long!

Give your nails the attention they deserve

Let's face it, we are all a sucker for pretty nails. There's just something about those beauties that all of us would love to have, regardless of the damage it really does.

If you have been one of the nail lovers through the months, odds are it's time to do your nails a little service and pay them the attention they deserve. Mix ½ cup Epsom salt with 1 teaspoon vitamin E oil and 1 teaspoon coconut oil in warm water. Keep the mixture thick enough that it's more of a paste than anything.

Use a Q-tip to spread the paste over your nails, and let sit for 20 minutes. Rinse off with warm water, and let your nails go nude for a while. Repeat every few days, and enjoy stronger, longer, and healthier nails!

Chapter 4 – Healthier Matters

So many times when you learn how to take care of your appearance naturally you are thrilled enough, but to know that you can use the same thing to take care of a variety of health issues makes this the perfect substance to have on hand for all of your needs.

I know that many of the ways you have been told to use Epsom salt revolve around soaking in the tub, but that is just the tip of the ice burg. I want you to know all the ways you can use this wonderful mineral, from putting it on your food to using it with the essential oils for the greatest benefit.

There's no way you can go wrong when you are using all natural ingredients, and with this one on hand, it doesn't matter what is headed your way, you have it covered.

Take a look at these all natural remedies for your health. You may be surprised at just how many ways you can use this in and on your body, and discover the rich benefits that come from using it often. If you want that extra bit of a boost, feel free to add in essential oils on top of it. The more natural you can go, with the more potent the ingredients, the better off you are going to be as a whole.

Keep your blood sugar under control easily

If you have diabetes, or if you are at risk for developing diabetes, you know what it means to be careful of salt intake. But, you are also well aware of having to watch how you eat and what you do in your day, because you have to also be careful of your blood sugar.

With Epsom salt, you have a new way to control and manage your blood sugar, and you can manage it without a lot of effort. Simply use the bath soak method, or try taking Epsom salt orally for the greatest results.

If you are going to take it orally, you simply have to sprinkle a bit on your dinner as you would regular table salt, and you will gain more benefits than you ever thought you would.

Relieve constipation without taking any pills

As surprising as it is, you can completely relieve any constipation you have within a single day with nothing more than a teaspoon of Epsom salt and some warm water. Simply dissolve the salt in the water and drink, then feel like your old self once again.

It is important that you take note this remedy can be overdone, and you should limit this to only once per day. Also, if you continue to have this problem for more than just a few days, you should get it checked out by a physician.

Relax your muscles much deeper than you thought you could

Of course you are aware that you can soak in an Epsom salt bath to relieve aches and pains, but did you know that you can use Epsom salt soaks to reduce the swelling of sprains, and heal bruises?

That's right, by mixing 1 cup of salt in a bowl of warm water and soaking the affected area, you are going to drastically reduce the swelling on any sprain, and nearly heal a bruise in a fraction of the time. Not only is this a relaxing way to spend your time, but you are going to cure those annoyances that like to slow you down.

It's the best of both worlds in one little remedy.

Get back on your feet in no time at all

I already outlined how you can use Epsom salt to take care of your nails, and of course you know that means your nails on your toes, too. But, you should know that this doesn't stop at just saving your nails from acrylics, but you can also get rid of athlete's foot and other fungal infections with Epsom salt, too.

Place 1/3 cup of Epsom salt in a bowl of warm water, and soak one foot in at a time. Let each foot soak for about 20 minutes to half and hour, and if you are currently dealing with fungal infections, you will see them clear up within days.

This is also an excellent way to prevent any future fungal infections from forming in the first place.

Ease gout and arthritis pain while you relax

Whether you need to do an entire body soak to ease the pain in your muscles or if you are going to stick with soaking just your hands or feet, you can relieve ailments such as gout and arthritis with your Epsom salt.

Again, all you need is the salt and a bit of warm water, combined in a bowl. Of course, I also recommend you use essential oils with this, as there are so many benefits to essential oils, but that is entirely up to you.

With regular soaking, you are going to eradicate the issues you had with gout, and you are going to have to take less arthritis medication. It's the best of both worlds in a bowl.

Whether you are looking for ways to take care of your muscles and joints to ways you can take care of your skin and hair, you are going to get them with Epsom salt.

But, there are still more good things to come, so don't feel like you have reached the end of the line yet. In the next chapter, I am going to show you some unconventional ways you can use Epsom salt around the house... this is going to not only help keep your home fresh and clean, but it will also keep dangerous chemicals away from your family where they belong.

Chapter 5 – All Natural Epsom Healing for the Home

I could go on to say how much Epsom salt is going to help your blood circulation, your stress levels, your digestive system, and even your heart, but I think you have gotten the idea by now. Clearly, this is the salt you want to have on hand at all times, and there is an obvious reason it has stood the test of time.

But, there are still more great uses you can indulge in when you are using Epsom salt, and those come in around the house. In this chapter, I want to show you all the wonderful ways you can use Epsom salt around your home, around your pets, and around your children without worry that you are exposing them to dangerous chemicals.

We all know the search for natural cleaners is one that will wage on, but this is your chance to use something that actually works in ways you never thought of before. Whether you are using it to keep your home clean, using it to rid your house of some of the more annoying guests you don't want around, or using it to deep clean parts of your house that haven't been done in a while, you are going to find what you need with this chapter.

Go ahead and indulge a little. If you want to add even more cleaning power, throw in some essential oils. There's no end to the ways you can make your home fresh and clean without using a single toxic chemical.

Your cleaning routine just got a little bit sweeter.

Deep clean your tile naturally... even with pets

For pet owners everywhere, it can be a real challenge to deep clean anything in your home. You have to worry about the chemicals around the animals, and you have to keep track of where they are and what they are doing while you try to work.

With this being said, it can be nearly impossible to deep clean any surface in your home. But, with Epsom salt, you have the freedom to clean anything you wish without worry that they are going to be in danger of any harmful chemicals.

Simply combine 2 cups of salt with warm water, or even add it to your normal cleaning agent, and scrub away. Not only is the abrasiveness going to clean the cracks, but you are going to kill germs and polish as you go... all without worry that you are exposing your furry friends to anything they shouldn't be around.

A total win for everyone.

Use Epsom salt to rid yourself of any pests you don't want around the home

Do you have unwanted ants crawling about? Do you have slugs in the garden? Do you have an issue with bugs around the walls and on the floor? While this may be a common issue a lot of people have to deal with, it's not anything you want to deal with in your home, and Epsom salt can help.

Again, you don't have to worry about exposing any of your furry friends to anything you don't want them to be around, and at the same time, you don't have to worry about the intruders coming back. Generously spray over any cracks in your home whenever you see ants or anything else gathering, and mix some salt in with your garden soil, and say goodbye to the pests at once!

Deep clean your drains and washers

You would be surprised at how much soap and detergents build up in your washer and drains over time. With Epsom salt, you can make a warm water solution and pour them down your drain or run them through your washer.

Depending on how long it's been, you might have to run more than one cycle to get everything clean, but you are going to be pleasantly surprised at how well this does the first time around.

I prefer to add 1 cup of Epsom salt to hot water and let this sit in my drain for an hour or so, then letting it drain completely. If I am using it in my washers, I like to add 1 cup of Epsom salt to the drum directly, then run a wash cycle with nothing else in it.

Let soak, and run the rinse, and that's it. Your drains are going to flush and all of your clothes will be cleaner.

Use Epsom salt in your dish water, especially when you have greasy or grimy dishes

If you are using a dish washer, use Epsom salt in the rinse water before you place it in the dishwasher. If you are washing by hand, sprinkle a generous amount in your sink before you wash your dishes, and scrub.

If you use the crystals in the sponge you will get greater scrubbing power, but this is up to you.

For particularly hard stains or baked on food, soak the dishes in an Epsom salt back for an hour or so before you wash... the food will wash right off!

Really, any cleaning you need done around the house you can do with Epsom salt, and you can do it all without worry that your pets or children are going to be around harmful chemicals or things you wish they weren't.

The more natural you can keep your home, the better off it's going to be for everyone, so go ahead, and by a large bag of Epsom salt today. You can find it at most health food stores, grocery stores, or even some department stores.

Remember that there is a reason this has lasted the test of time, and so many people across the globe have used it for a variety of ailments and illness. Now, it's your turn. Use Epsom salt for anything and everything you need, and you will see the benefits come rolling in.

Conclusion

There you have it, everything you need to know to use Epsom salt as your miracle cure, and how to use it to take care of all your health and beauty needs. I know when you are first starting out something like this, you can be a little skeptical. But with this book, you are going to find everything you need to know about this incredible mineral, and discover just how many ways you can use it for your health.

If you are careful to follow all of the tips and tricks in this book, you are going to discover so many ways this mineral can heal you. It doesn't matter what you are dealing with, this salt is just what you need to cure, revitalize, and shine!

Let me show you the secrets you need to truly embracing your health, and diving into a world like you have never known before. This book has everything you need to gain better health, and with it, you are going to achieve that energetic and happy lifestyle you have always wanted.

So turn back the clocks and say goodbye to the stress. You have found a miracle solution that is better than all the rest. Rest easy knowing that you are going to get the best results you can imagine using this mineral, and say goodbye to the wrinkles, aches, and pains.

Join the millions of people who have been using this wonderful mineral for centuries, and let the relief rush in.

FREE Bonus Reminder

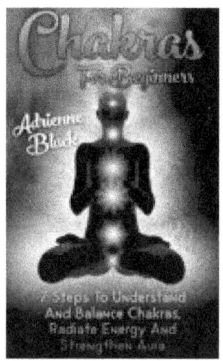

If you have not grabbed it yet, please go ahead and download your special bonus E book *"Chakras for Beginners. 7 Steps To Understand And Balance Chakras, Radiate Energy, And Strengthen Aura"*.

Simply Click the Button Below

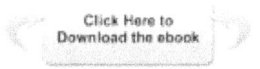

OR Go to This Page

http://lifehacksworld.com/free

BONUS #2: More Free & Discounted Books & Products

Do you want to receive more Free/Discounted Books or Products?

We have a mailing list where we send out our new Books or Products when they go free or with a discount on Amazon. Click on the link below to sign up for Free & Discount Book & Product Promotions.

=> Sign Up for Free & Discount Book & Product Promotions <=

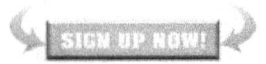

OR Go to this URL

http://zbit.ly/1WBb1Ek

www.ingramcontent.com/pod-product-compliance
Lightning Source LLC
Chambersburg PA
CBHW072012280526
45788CB00005B/2014